certain other noncommercial uses

permitted by copyright law

# Contents

# Get Your Vitamin P: Why Pleasure Matters When It Comes to What You Eat

Nearly everyone has an answer to the question 'what's your favorite food?.'

It's easy to see why: humans are wired to derive pleasure from food. In fact, for many, eating ranks among the greatest pleasures in life!

Besides making mealtimes an enjoyable experience, taking pleasure from food also has significant benefits for health. Savoring food supports digestion, can help improve your relationship with food, can help overcome disordered eating and more.

In some cases, getting enough "vitamin P" (or perhaps vitamin mmmm) is just as important as the contents of your plate. Read on to dive into the tasty delights of why pleasure matters for food.

## The psychology behind eating for pleasure

For years, researchers have studied the science behind eating for pleasure. Their findings are intriguing and largely encouraging.

Physiologically, the pleasure people derive from food occurs both in our mouths and in our brains.

"Pleasure of any kind, including pleasure from food, leads to a release of dopamine in the brain," explains therapist, dietitian, and Certified Body Trust provider Aleta Storch, RDN, MHC, of Wise Heart Nutrition and Wellness.

"Dopamine is often referred to as the 'feel good hormone' because it activates the reward pathways in the brain, which helps to promote happiness, calmness, motivation, and focus," she says.

In fact, some older 2011 researchTrusted Source indicates that people with obesity may have disrupted dopamine sensitivity, leading them to overeat to achieve adequate pleasure from food.

When brain chemistry is working properly, however, our enjoyment of food can lead to physical benefits.

"When we enjoy the food we are eating and stimulate dopamine, we actually digest and metabolize it more effectively," says Storch. "When we're relaxed in response to having a pleasurable eating experience, our nervous system goes into rest and digest mode, which allows us to fully break down and utilize the nutrients from the foods we eat."

Eating for pleasure could promote healthier eating too.

A review examined 119 studies about the connection between food enjoyment and a healthy diet. Fifty-seven percent of the studies found favorable associations between eating pleasure and dietary outcomes.

for example, associated greater eating pleasure with higher nutritional status. Others have emphasized the importance of taking pleasure from healthy foods to promote a nourishing, balanced diet.

"There's this belief that 'healthy' food has to be bland or it doesn't taste good, but that's just not true," says dietitian and certified intuitive eating counselor Sarah Gold Anzlovar, MS, RDN, LDN. "When we eat food that we enjoy, satisfaction increases, which can actually improve diet quality and reduce the chance of overeating or binge episodes."

The emotional nourishment of the foods we eat

Mealtimes would be pretty boring if food was just fuel. Eating casts a wide net across the human experience, from bringing us together with loved ones to connecting us to our cultural heritage.

In short, food is emotional as well as physical nourishment. Here are some of the ways enjoying food can feed your spirit.

Food enjoyment increases social connection

What's a party or family gathering without something to munch on?

As people enjoy meals with others, it often contributes to an increased sense of happiness, according to a study on Thai social communities.

Food enjoyment offers physical and emotional comfort

Warm chicken soup when you're sick, a pasta that reminds you of your grandmother, or the favorite dessert that always seems to hit the spot: foods like these have a way of lifting our spirits and soothing our bodies.

"Sometimes food even offers comfort at the end of a challenging day, which many people associate as negative emotional eating," says Anzlovar. "But when we allow ourselves to connect with the food and enjoy it, there are many benefits."

Food enjoyment breaks the hold of diet culture

Diet culture has multiple definitions, but one hallmark of this societal-level messaging is that you have to say no to foods you love, especially if they're high in calories or fat.

Choosing to mindfully enjoy what you eat helps break this harmful mentality.

"When all foods are allowed without rules—including the most delicious ones, the body learns to trust that it will get what it needs," says Storch."Creating permission for these foods that have been labeled as 'bad' or 'off-limits' is an important step in the healing process, and can help someone to feel more peace, confidence, and freedom around food."

Food enjoyment connects us with our cultural heritage

For decades, study has demonstrated that a sense of belonging is vital to mental health. What more beautiful place to experience belonging than within your family or cultural heritage?

Here's where food enjoyment could play a major role.

"Culture and tradition serve as a form of connection with others and ourselves," says

Storch. "Restricting or denying foods that promote connection can lead to disengagement and loneliness. By omitting cultural foods, we are saying not only that the food is 'bad' but that the underlying identity associated with the food is 'bad.'"

Embracing these foods could ultimately create a sense of freedom and belonging that elevate your mental health.

Eating for pleasure vs. emotional eating

You've probably heard that emotional eating isn't ideal.

Turning to food to deal with difficult emotions like stress, anger, or sadness often results in mindless consumption and creates a fraught relationship with food. That said, it's understandable if you're wary of the idea of eating for pleasure.

Fortunately, emotional eating and eating for pleasure differ in both their intent and their outcomes.

"Emotional eating is when people are using food as a way to cope with both positive or negative emotions," says Anzlovar. "Eating for pleasure is choosing a food to specifically enjoy its taste, texture, and experience, such as when you go out for an ice cream cone in the summer or eat an apple straight from the tree at an apple orchard."

Another major distinction between these two behaviors is the connection you feel toward your food.

"Often, though not always, there is a lack of connection or disassociation with the food when people emotionally eat," Anzlovar explains. "When eating for pleasure, there's usually a true connection and enjoyment that you are getting from the food."

Of course, there's no perfectly drawn line between emotional eating and eating for enjoyment—and sometimes the two may overlap.

One way to tell which you're practicing: How do you feel afterward?

Making a point to mindfully enjoy your food won't leave you with feelings of guilt or shame.

# Introduction

## What is a Balanced Diet?

A balanced diet is one that provides the body with all the essential nutrients it needs to stay healthy. It is made up of a variety of foods from different food groups, such as grains, fruits, vegetables, dairy, protein, and fats. Eating a balanced diet ensures that you get all the vitamins and minerals your body needs to function properly.

## Benefits of Eating a Balanced Diet

Eating a balanced diet has many benefits, such as:

- Improved physical health: Eating a balanced diet can help you maintain a healthy weight and reduce your risk of certain diseases, such as heart disease, diabetes, and some cancers.

- Improved mental health: Eating a balanced diet can help reduce stress and improve mood.

• Increased energy: Eating a balanced diet can help you feel more energized throughout the day.

• Improved cognitive function: Eating a balanced diet can help improve your memory, focus, and concentration.

• Improved digestion: Eating a balanced diet can help promote regularity and improve digestion.

# Macronutrients

## Carbohydrates

Carbohydrates are the body's primary source of energy. They are found in foods such as grains, fruits, vegetables, and legumes. Eating a variety of carbohydrates can provide the body with the energy it needs to function properly.

## Fats

Fats are an important part of a healthy diet. They provide the body with energy, support cell growth, and help the body absorb certain vitamins. Fats can be found in foods such as nuts, seeds, avocados, olive oil, and fish.

## Section A: Grains

Grains are a type of carbohydrate that provide energy and fiber to the body. Examples of grains include wheat, rice, oats, barley, quinoa, and corn. Eating a variety of grains, such as whole grains, can help provide essential vitamins and minerals, such as iron and B vitamins.

## Section B: Fruits

Fruits are a type of carbohydrate that provide energy, fiber, vitamins, and minerals. Examples of fruits include apples, oranges, bananas, grapes, strawberries, and blueberries. Eating a variety of fruits can help provide essential nutrients and promote overall health.

## Section C: Vegetables

Vegetables are a type of carbohydrate that provide energy, fiber, vitamins, and minerals. Examples of vegetables include leafy greens, carrots, tomatoes, peppers, and potatoes. Eating a variety of vegetables is important for overall health and can help reduce the risk of certain diseases.

## Section D: Dairy

Dairy is a type of food that provides protein, calcium, and vitamins. Examples of dairy include milk, cheese, yogurt, and butter. Eating dairy can help promote strong bones and teeth, as well as provide essential vitamins and minerals.

## Section E: Protein

Protein is an essential nutrient that provides energy, helps build and repair body tissue, and helps maintain healthy bones and muscles. Examples of protein include lean meats, poultry, fish, eggs, beans, and nuts. Eating a variety of proteins can help provide essential nutrients and promote overall health.

# Balanced Diet

## What is a balanced diet?

A balanced diet gives your body the nutrients it needs to function correctly. To get the nutrition you need, most of your daily calories should come from:

- fresh fruits

- fresh vegetables

- whole grains

- legumes

- nuts

- lean proteins

The Dietary Guidelines for AmericansTrusted Source explain how much of each nutrient you should consume daily.

## About calories

The number of calories in a food refers to the amount of energy stored in that food. Your body uses calories from food for walking, thinking, breathing, and other important functions.

The average person needs about 2,000 calories every day to maintain their weight, but the amount will depend on their age, sex, and physical activity level.

Males tend to need more calories than females, and people who exercise need more calories than people who don't.

Current guidelines list the following calorie intakes for males and females of different ages:

## Person Calorie requirements

Sedentary children: 2–8 years 1,000–1,400

Active children: 2–8 years 1,000–2,000

Females: 9–13 years 1,400–2,200

Males: 9–13 years 1,600–2,600

Active females: 14–30 years 2,400

Sedentary females: 14–30 years 1,800–2,000

Active males: 14–30 years 2,800–3,200

Sedentary males: 14–30 years 2,000–2,600

Active people: 30 years and over 2,000–3,000

Sedentary people: 30 years and over 1,600–2,400

The source of your daily calories are also important. Foods that provide mainly calories and very little nutrition are known as "empty calories."

Examples of foods that provide empty calories include:

- cakes, cookies, and donuts

- processed meats

- energy drinks and sodas

- fruit drinks with added sugar

- ice cream

- chips and fries

- pizza

- sodas

However, it's not only the type of food but the ingredients that make it nutritious.

A homemade pizza with a wholemeal base and plenty of fresh veggies on top may be a healthy choice. In contrast, premade pizzas and other highly processed foods often contain empty calories.

To maintain good health, limit your consumption of empty calories and instead try to get your calories from foods that are rich in other nutrients.

Why a balanced diet is important

A balanced diet supplies the nutrients your body needs to work effectively. Without balanced nutrition, your body is more prone to disease, infection, fatigue, and low performance.

Children who don't get enough healthy foods may face growth and developmental problems, poor academic performance, and frequent infections.

They can also develop unhealthy eating habits that may persist into adulthood.

Without exercise, they'll also have a higher risk of obesity and various diseases that make up metabolic syndrome, such as type 2 diabetes and high blood pressure.

According to the Center for Science in the Public Interest, 4 of the top 10 leading causes of death in the United States are directly linked to diet.

These are:

- heart disease

- cancer

- stroke

- type 2 diabetes

## SUMMARY

Your body needs nutrients to stay healthy, and food supplies essential nutrients that stop us from getting sick.

What to eat for a balanced diet

A healthy, balanced diet will usually include the following nutrients:

• vitamins, minerals, and antioxidants

• carbohydrates, including starches and fiber

• protein

• healthy fats

A balanced diet will include a variety of foods from the following groups:

• fruits

• vegetables

- grains

- dairy

- protein foods

Examples of protein foods include meat, eggs, fish, beans, nuts, and legumes.

People who follow a vegan diet will focus entirely on plant-based foods. They won't eat meat, fish, or dairy, but their diet will include other items that provide similar nutrients.

Tofu and beans, for example, are plant-based sources of protein. Some people are intolerant of dairy but can still build a balanced diet by choosing a variety of nutrient-rich replacements.

## Foods to avoid

Foods to avoid or limit on a healthy diet include:

- highly processed foods

- refined grains

- added sugar and salt

- red and processed meat

- alcohol

- trans fats

What's healthy for one person may not be suitable for another.

Whole wheat flour can be a healthy ingredient for many people but isn't suitable for those with a gluten intolerance, for example.

## Fruits

Fruits are nutritious, they make a tasty snack or dessert, and they can satisfy a sweet tooth.

Local fruits that are in season are fresher and provide more nutrients than imported fruits.

Fruits are high in sugar, but this sugar is natural. Unlike candies and many sweet desserts, fruits also provide fiber and other nutrients. This means they're less likely to cause a sugar spike and they'll boost the body's supply of essential vitamins, minerals, and antioxidants.

If you have diabetes, your doctor or dietitian can advise you on which fruits to choose, how much to eat, and when.

# Vegetables

Vegetables are a key source of essential vitamins, minerals, and antioxidants. Eat a variety of vegetables with different colors for a full range of nutrients.

Dark, leafy greens are an excellent source of many nutrients. They include:

- spinach

- kale

- green beans

- broccoli

- collard greens

• Swiss chard

Local, seasonal vegetables are often reasonable in price and easy to prepare. Use them in the following ways:

• as a side dish

• roasted in a tray with a splash of olive oil

• as the base in soups, stews, and pasta dishes

• as a salad

• in purées

• in juices and smoothies

# Grains

Refined white flour is featured in many breads and baked goods, but it has limited nutritional value. This is because much of the goodness is in the hull of the grain, or outer shell, which manufacturers remove during processing.

Whole grain products include the entire grain, including the hull. They provide additional vitamins, minerals, and fiber. Many people also find that whole grains add flavor and texture to a dish.

Try switching from white breads, pastas, and rice to whole grain options.

# Proteins

Meats and beans are primary sources of protein, which is essential for wound healing and muscle maintenance and development, among other functions.

## Animal protein

Healthy animal-based options include:

- red meats, such as beef and mutton

- poultry, such as chicken and turkey

- fish, including salmon, sardines, and other oily fish

Processed meats and red meats may increase the risk of cancer and other diseases, according to some.

Some processed meats also contain a lot of added preservatives and salt. Fresh, unprocessed meat is the best option.

## Plant-based protein

Nuts, beans, and soy products are good sources of protein, fiber, and other nutrients.

Examples include:

- lentils

- beans

- peas

- almonds

- sunflower seeds

- walnuts

Tofu, tempeh, and other soy-based products are excellent sources of protein and are healthy alternatives to meat.

## Dairy

Dairy products provide essential nutrients, including:

- protein

- calcium

- vitamin D

They also contain fat. If you're seeking to limit your fat intake, reduced fat options might be best. Your doctor can help you decide.

For those following a vegan diet, many dairy-free milks and other dairy alternatives are now available, made from:

- flax seed

- almonds and cashews

- soy

- oats

- coconut

These are often fortified with calcium and other nutrients, making them excellent alternatives to dairy from cows. Some have added sugar, so read the label carefully when choosing.

Shop for almond and soy milk.

## Fats and oils

Fat is essential for energy and cell health, but too much fat can increase calories above what the body needs and may lead to weight gain.

In the past, guidelines have recommended avoiding saturated fats, due to concerns that they would raise cholesterol levels.

More recent research suggests that partially replacing with unsaturated fats lowers cardiovascular disease risk and that some saturated fat should remain in the diet — about 10 percent or less of calories.

Trans fats, however, should still be avoided.

Recommendations on fats can sometimes be hard to follow, but one scientistTrusted Source has proposed the following guideline:

• Fats to love: vegetable oils and fish oils

- Fats to limit: butter, cheese, and heavy cream

- Fats to lose: trans fats, used in many processed and premade foods, such as donuts

Most experts consider olive oil to be a healthy fat, and especially extra virgin olive oil, which is the least processed type.

Deep fried foods are often high in calories but low in nutritional value, so you should eat them sparingly.

SUMMARY

A balanced diet contains foods from the following groups: fruits, vegetables, dairy, grains, and protein.

## Putting it all together

A healthy diet will combine all the nutrients and foods groups mentioned above, but you need to balance them, too.

A handy way to remember how much of each food group to eat is the plate method. The USDA's "ChooseMyPlate" initiative recommends:

- filling half your plate with fruits and vegetables

- filling just over one quarter with grains

- filling just under one quarter with protein foods

- adding dairy on the side (or a nondairy replacement)

But individual needs will vary, so the USDA also provides an interactive tool, "MyPlate Plan" where you can enter your own details to find out your personal needs.

SUMMARY

Aim for around half your food to come from fruits and vegetables, around one quarter to be protein, and one quarter whole grains and starches.

Bottom line

A varied and healthy diet is usually one that contains plenty of fresh, plant-based foods, and limits the intake of processed foods.

If you have questions about your diet or feel that you need to lose weight or change your eating habits, schedule an appointment with your doctor or a dietitian.

They can suggest dietary changes that will help you get the nutrition you need while promoting your overall health.

# 50 Foods That Are Super Healthy

It's easy to wonder which foods are healthiest.

A vast number of foods are both healthy and tasty. By filling your plate with fruits, vegetables, quality protein, and other whole foods, you'll have meals that are colorful, versatile, and good for you.

Here are 50 incredibly healthy foods. Most of them are surprisingly delicious.

# 1–6: Fruits and berries

Fruits and berries are among the world's most popular health foods.

These sweet, nutritious foods are very easy to incorporate into your diet because they require little to no preparation.

# 1. Apples

Apples are high in fiber, vitamin C, and numerous antioxidants. They are very filling and make the perfect snack if you find yourself hungry between meals.

## 2. Avocados

Avocados are different than most fruits because they are loaded with healthy fats instead of carbs. Not only are they creamy and tasty but also high in fiber, potassium, and vitamin C.

## 3. Bananas

Bananas are among the world's best sources of potassium. They're also high in vitamin B6 and fiber, as well as convenient and portable.

# 4. Blueberries

Blueberries are not only delicious but also among the most powerful sources of antioxidants in the world.

# 5. Oranges

Oranges are well known for their vitamin C content. What's more, they're high in fiber and antioxidants.

6. Strawberries

Strawberries are highly nutritious and low in both carbs and calories.

They are loaded with vitamin C, fiber, and manganese and are arguably among the most delicious foods in existence.

Other healthy fruits

Other health fruits and berries include cherries, grapes, grapefruit, kiwifruit, lemons, mango, melons, olives, peaches, pears, pineapples, plums, and raspberries.

7. Eggs

Eggs are among the most nutritious foods on the planet.

They were previously demonized for being high in cholesterol, but new studies show that they're perfectly safe and healthy.

## 8–10: Meats

Unprocessed, gently cooked meat is one of the most nutritious foods you can eat.

### 8. Lean beef

Lean beef is among the best sources of protein in existence and loaded with highly bioavailable iron. Choosing the fatty cuts is fine if you're on a low-carb diet.

### 9. Chicken breasts

Chicken breast is low in fat and calories but extremely high in protein. It's a great source of many nutrients. Again, feel free to eat fattier cuts of chicken if you're not eating that many carbs.

10. Lamb

Lambs are usually grass-fed, and their meat tends to be high in omega-3 fatty acids.

11–15: Nuts and seeds

Despite being high in fat and calories, nuts and seeds may help you lose weight.

These foods are crunchy, filling, and loaded with important nutrients that many people don't get enough of, including magnesium and vitamin E.

They also require almost no preparation, so they're easy to add to your routine.

## 11. Almonds

Almonds are a popular nut loaded with vitamin E, antioxidants, magnesium, and fiber. Studies show that almonds can help you lose weight and improve metabolic health.

## 12. Chia seeds

Chia seeds are among the most nutrient-dense foods on the planet. A single ounce

(28 grams) packs 11 grams of fiber and significant amounts of magnesium, manganese, calcium, and various other nutrients.

## 13. Coconuts

Coconuts are loaded with fiber and powerful fatty acids called medium-chain triglycerides (MCTs).

## 14. Macadamia nuts

Macadamia nuts are very tasty. They're much higher in monounsaturated fats and lower in omega-6 fatty acids than most other nuts.

## 15. Walnuts

Walnuts are highly nutritious and loaded with fiber and various vitamins and minerals.

## 16–25: Vegetables

Calorie for calorie, vegetables are among the world's most concentrated sources of nutrients.

There's a wide variety available, and it's best to eat many different types every day.

## 16. Asparagus

Asparagus is a popular vegetable. It's low in both carbs and calories but loaded with vitamin K.

## 17. Bell peppers

Bell peppers come in several colors, including red, yellow, and green. They're crunchy and sweet, as well as a great source of antioxidants and vitamin C.

## 18. Broccoli

Broccoli is a cruciferous vegetable that tastes great both raw and cooked. It's an excellent source of fiber and vitamins C and K and contains a decent amount of protein compared with other vegetables.

## 19. Carrots

Carrots are a popular root vegetable. They are extremely crunchy and loaded with nutrients like fiber and vitamin K.

Carrots are also very high in carotene antioxidants, which have numerous benefits.

## 20. Cauliflower

Cauliflower is a very versatile cruciferous vegetable. It can be used to make a multitude of healthy dishes — and also tastes good on its own.

## 21. Cucumber

Cucumbers are one of the world's most popular vegetables. They're very low in both carbs and calories, consisting mostly of water. However, they contain a number of nutrients in small amounts, including vitamin K.

## 22. Garlic

Garlic is incredibly healthy. It contains bioactive organosulfur compounds that have powerful biological effects, including improved immune function .

## 23. Kale

Kale has become increasingly popular because it's incredibly high in fiber, vitamins

C and K, and a number of other nutrients. It adds a satisfying crunch to salads and other dishes.

## 24. Onions

Onions have a very strong flavor and are very popular in many recipes. They contain a number of bioactive compounds believed to have health benefits.

## 25. Tomatoes

Tomatoes are usually categorized as a vegetable, although they are technically a fruit. They are tasty and loaded with nutrients like potassium and vitamin C.

More healthy vegetables

Most vegetables are very healthy. Others worth mentioning include artichokes, Brussels sprouts, cabbage, celery, eggplant, leeks, lettuce, mushrooms, radishes, squash, Swiss chard, turnips, and zucchini.

26–31: Fish and seafood

Fish and other seafood tend to be very healthy and nutritious.

They're especially rich in omega-3 fatty acids and iodine, two nutrients in which most people are deficient.

Studies show that people who eat the highest amounts of seafood — especially fish — tend to live longer and have a lower risk of many illnesses, including heart disease, dementia, and depression ( 9Trusted Source, 10, 11).

26. Salmon

Salmon is a type of oily fish that's incredibly popular due to its excellent taste and high amount of nutrients, including protein and omega-3 fatty acids. It also contains some vitamin D.

27. Sardines

Sardines are small, oily fish that are among the most nutritious foods you can eat. They boast sizable amounts of most nutrients that your body needs.

28. Shellfish

Shellfish ranks similarly to organ meats when it comes to nutrient density. Edible shellfish include clams, mollusks, and oysters.

29. Shrimp

Shrimp is a type of crustacean related to crabs and lobsters. It tends to be low in fat and calories but high in protein. It's also loaded with various other nutrients, including selenium and vitamin B12.

30. Trout

Trout is another type of delicious freshwater fish, similar to salmon.

31. Tuna

Tuna is very popular in Western countries and tends to be low in fat and calories while high in protein. It's perfect for people who need to add more protein to their diets but keep calories low.

However, you should make sure to buy low-mercury varieties.

## 32–34: Grains

Although grains have gotten a bad rap in recent years, some types are very healthy.

Just keep in mind that they're relatively high in carbs, so they're not recommended for a low-carb diet.

## 32. Brown rice

Rice is one of the most popular cereal grains and is currently a staple food for more than half of the world's population. Brown rice is fairly nutritious, with a decent amount of fiber, vitamin B1, and magnesium.

## 33. Oats

Oats are incredibly healthy. They are loaded with nutrients and powerful fibers called beta glucans, which provide numerous benefits.

## 34. Quinoa

Quinoa has become incredibly popular among health-conscious individuals in recent years. It's a tasty grain that's high in nutrients, such as fiber and magnesium. It is also an excellent source of plant-based protein.

## 35–36: Breads

Many people eat a lot of highly processed white bread.

For those trying to adopt a healthier diet, it can be extremely challenging to find healthy breads. Even so, options are available.

## 35. Ezekiel bread

Ezekiel bread may be the healthiest bread you can buy. It's made from organic, sprouted whole grains, as well as several legumes.

## 36. Homemade low-carb breads

Overall, the best choice for bread may be that which you can make yourself.

## 37–40: Legumes

Legumes are another food group that has been unfairly demonized.

While it's true that legumes contain antinutrients, which can interfere with digestion and absorption of nutrients, they can be eliminated by soaking and proper preparation.

Therefore, legumes are a great plant-based source of protein.

37. Green beans

Green beans, also called string beans, are unripe varieties of the common bean. They are very popular in Western countries.

## 38. Kidney beans

Kidney beans are loaded with fiber and various vitamins and minerals. Make sure to cook them properly, as they're toxic when raw.

## 39. Lentils

Lentils are another popular legume. They're high in fiber and among the best sources of plant-based protein.

## 40. Peanuts

Peanuts (which are legumes, not a true nuts) are incredibly tasty and high in nutrients and antioxidants. Several studies suggest that peanuts can help you lose weight.

However, take it easy on the peanut butter, as it's very high in calories and easy to overeat.

41–43: Dairy

For those who can tolerate them, dairy products are a healthy source of various important nutrients.

Full-fat dairy seems to be the best, and studies show that people who eat the most full-fat dairy have a lower risk of obesity and type 2 diabetes.

If the dairy comes from grass-fed cows, it may be even more nutritious — as it's higher in some bioactive fatty acids like conjugated linoleic acid (CLA) and vitamin K2.

41. Cheese

Cheese is incredibly nutritious, as a single slice may offer about the same amount of nutrients as an entire cup (240 ml) of milk. For many, it's also one of the most delicious foods you can eat.

42. Whole milk

Whole milk is very high in vitamins, minerals, quality animal protein, and healthy fats. What's more, it's one of the best dietary sources of calcium.

## 43. Yogurt

Yogurt is made from milk that's fermented by adding live bacteria to it. It has many of the same health effects as milk, but yogurt with live cultures has the added benefit of friendly probiotic bacteria.

## 44–46: Fats and oils

Many fats and oils are now marketed as health foods, including several sources of saturated fat that were previously demonized.

## 44. Butter from grass-fed cows

Butter from grass-fed cows is high in many important nutrients, including vitamin K2.

## 45. Coconut oil

Coconut oil contains relatively high amounts of MCTs, may aid Alzheimer's disease, and has been shown to help you lose belly fat.

## 46. Extra virgin olive oil

Extra virgin olive oil is one of the healthiest vegetable oils you can find. It contains heart-healthy monounsaturated fats and is very high in antioxidants with powerful health benefits.

## 47–48: Tubers

Tubers are the storage organs of some plants. They tend to contain a number of beneficial nutrients.

## 47. Potatoes

Potatoes are loaded with potassium and contain a little bit of almost every nutrient you need, including vitamin C.

They'll also keep you full for long periods. One study analyzed 38 foods and found that boiled potatoes were by far the most filling.

## 48. Sweet potatoes

Sweet potatoes are among the most delicious starchy foods you can eat. They're loaded with antioxidants and all sorts of healthy nutrients.

## 49. Apple cider vinegar

Apple cider vinegar is incredibly popular in the natural health community. Studies show that it can help lower blood sugar levels and cause modest weight loss.

It's great to use as a salad dressing or to add flavor to meals.

## 50. Dark chocolate

Dark chocolate is loaded with magnesium and serves as one of the planet's most powerful sources of antioxidants (20).

The bottom line

Whether you want to overhaul your diet or simply change up your meals, it's easy to add a number of these foods to your routine.

Many of the foods above not only make a great snack but are also packed with vitamins and antioxidants. Some of them may even aid weight loss.

If you don't normally challenge your palate, don't be afraid of trying something new.